# Simple Understanding of Lupus SLE

*Lupus SLE: Essential Insights and Understanding*

**LK Weston**

*To my loving children, Mysti Kay, Brandee Kay, and Dalene Kay,*

*This book is dedicated to all of you, my eternal source of strength and inspiration. Through the uncertainties and challenges posed by Lupus SLE, you have been my pillars of unwavering support, teaching me resilience, patience, and the true essence of unconditional love.*

*Your understanding, compassion, and boundless love have illuminated my darkest days, fueling my determination to navigate this journey with courage and hope. May this book serve as a testament to our enduring bond and as a guiding light for others facing similar battles.*

*With all my love, forever and always, Momma*

*"Understanding Lupus SLE is not solely about mastering its complexities, but finding strength in simplicity, empathy in knowledge, and hope in awareness."*

# Table of Contents

CHAPTER ONE

---

# *Understanding Lupus*

- **What is Systemic Lupus Erythematosus (SLE)?**

- **The Immune System and Lupus**

- **Causes and Risk Factors**

- **Common Symptoms and Signs**

### *Systemic Lupus Erythematosus (SLE)*

Systemic Lupus Erythematosus is a complex autoimmune disease. "It's when your body's immune system mistakenly attacks healthy tissues and organs. This immune system dysfunction can lead to inflammation and damage in various parts of the body. Lupus is known as a "systemic" disease because it can affect multiple systems or organs within the body, including the skin, joints, kidneys, heart, lungs, brain, and blood cells.

### *The Immune System and Lupus*

- The immune system plays a vital role in defending the body against harmful invaders such as bacteria, viruses, and other foreign substances. In a healthy immune system, a complex network of cells and proteins work together to recognize and destroy these invaders while leaving the body's own cells unharmed.

- In the case of lupus, something goes awry with the immune system. It produces autoantibodies—antibodies that target and attack the body's own cells and tissues. This leads to inflammation and tissue damage. The exact cause of this immune system malfunction is not fully understood, but a combination of genetic, environmental, and hormonal factors likely contributes to its development.

### *Causes and Risk Factors*

The precise cause of lupus remains unclear, but there are several factors that may increase an individual's risk of developing the disease. These factors include:

- Genetics: A family history of lupus or other autoimmune diseases can increase one's susceptibility to the condition.

- 

Hormones: Lupus is more common in women, particularly during their childbearing years. Hormonal factors may play a role, as hormonal changes can trigger or exacerbate symptoms.

- Environmental Triggers: Various environmental factors, such as exposure to sunlight, infections, certain medications, and stress, are thought to trigger or worsen lupus symptoms in genetically predisposed individuals.

### Common Symptoms and Signs

Lupus can manifest in a wide range of symptoms, and they can vary greatly from one individual to another. Common symptoms and signs of lupus include:

- Fatiguc: Extreme tiredness or weakness is a common complaint among people with lupus.

- Joint Pain and Swelling: Lupus often causes joint pain and swelling, similar to arthritis.

- Skin Rashes: A characteristic butterfly-shaped rash on the face, as well as other skin rashes, can occur in lupus patients.

- Photosensitivity: Many people with lupus are sensitive to sunlight and may develop skin rashes or other symptoms after sun exposure.

- 

Fever: Fever is a frequent symptom of lupus, often accompanying disease flares.

- Kidney Involvement: Lupus can damage the kidneys, leading to symptoms such as blood in the urine, high blood pressure, and kidney inflammation.

- Chest Pain and Breathing Problems: Inflammation of the heart or lungs can cause chest pain, breathing difficulties, and other cardiac or respiratory issues.

- Neurological Symptoms: Some people with lupus may experience neurological problems, including headaches, seizures, and cognitive difficulties.

- Blood Disorders: Lupus can affect blood cells, leading to anemia, a decreased number of platelets (which help with blood clotting), and an increased risk of blood clots.

It's important to note that lupus is a highly individualized disease, and not all individuals will experience the same symptoms. Diagnosis and management of lupus often require a careful evaluation by a healthcare professional, typically a rheumatologist, who specializes in autoimmune diseases. Treatment can involve medications to control symptoms and prevent flares, as well as lifestyle modifications to reduce triggers and improve overall well-being.

*A place to write down your questions, thoughts, and other notes:*

1. +

2. +

3. +

4. +

5. +

6. +

7. +

**"Believe in the beauty of your dreams and the power of your resilience;**

**for within you lies the strength to create a radiant tomorrow."**

**- Anonymous**

***

# CHAPTER 1 PERSONAL NOTES

CHAPTER TWO

---

# *Diagnosing Lupus*

- **The Diagnostic Process**

- **Medical Tests and Examinations**

- **The Role of Healthcare Providers**

- **Obtaining an Accurate Diagnosis**

Diagnosing lupus can be a complex process because its symptoms can mimic those of other diseases, and they often vary from person to person. This chapter will discuss the diagnostic process, the medical tests and examinations used in diagnosing lupus, the role of healthcare providers, and how to obtain an accurate diagnosis.

***The Diagnostic Process:***

The diagnostic process for lupus typically involves several steps. It begins with a thorough medical history and physical examination. Your healthcare provider will ask you about your symptoms, family history, and any other relevant medical information. They will then perform a physical examination to check for signs of lupus, such as skin rashes, joint swelling, or organ involvement.

### *Medical Tests and Examinations:*

Blood Tests: Various blood tests can help diagnose lupus. These include:

Antinuclear Antibody (ANA) Test: A positive ANA test is a common indicator of lupus, but it is not conclusive on its own.

- Complete Blood Count (CBC): This test can reveal low red blood cell counts (anemia) or low white blood cell counts (leukopenia), which are common in lupus.

- Erythrocyte Sedimentation Rate (ESR) and C-reactive Protein (CRP): Elevated levels of these markers can indicate inflammation.

- Autoantibody Tests: Tests for specific autoantibodies like anti-dsDNA, anti-Smith, and anti-phospholipid antibodies can help confirm a lupus diagnosis.

- Urinalysis: Checking for protein and blood in the urine is important as lupus can affect the kidneys.

- 

Imaging: X-rays, ultrasound, or other imaging tests may be used to examine affected organs or joints.

- Skin Biopsy: In cases of skin rashes, a small sample of skin may be taken for examination under a microscope to determine if it's related to lupus.

- Kidney and Biopsy: In cases of kidney involvement, a kidney biopsy may be performed to assess the extent of damage.

- Other Specialized Tests: Depending on your symptoms, additional tests like a chest X-ray, echocardiogram, or a lumbar puncture (spinal tap) may be necessary.

### The Role of Healthcare Providers:

Several healthcare providers may be involved in the diagnosis and management of lupus:

- Primary Care Physician: Your primary care doctor often initiates the diagnostic process and may refer you to specialists.

- Rheumatologist: These specialists focus on autoimmune diseases like lupus and play a central role in diagnosis and ongoing care.

- Dermatologist: If skin symptoms are prominent, a dermatologist may be consulted.

Nephrologist: For kidney involvement, a nephrologist may be involved.

- Other Specialists: Depending on affected organs or systems, other specialists like cardiologists, pulmonologists, or neurologists might be consulted.

### *Obtaining an Accurate Diagnosis:*

Obtaining an accurate diagnosis for lupus can be challenging, given its diverse and often overlapping symptoms. Here are some tips to ensure an accurate diagnosis:

- Be open and honest with your healthcare providers about your symptoms and medical history.

- Keep a symptom diary to record the frequency and severity of your symptoms.

- Seek a second opinion if you are uncertain about your diagnosis.

- Be patient, as diagnosing lupus can take time and may require multiple tests and consultations.

Remember that lupus is a complex and variable disease, and the diagnostic process may differ from person to person. Collaboration between you and your healthcare team is crucial in obtaining an accurate diagnosis and developing an appropriate treatment plan.

***A place to write down your questions, thoughts, and other notes:***

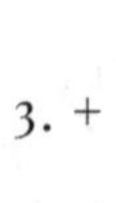

1. +

2. +

3. +

4. +

5. +

6. +

7. +

"Courage doesn't always roar. Sometimes courage is the quiet voice

at the end of the day saying, 'I will try again tomorrow.'"

- Mary Anne Radmacher

***

# CHAPTER 2 PERSONAL NOTES

CHAPTER THREE

# Types of Lupus

- **Systemic Lupus Erythematosus**

- **Cutaneous Lupus**

- **Drug-Induced Lupus**

- **Neonatal Lupus**

Lupus, or systemic lupus erythematosus (SLE), is a complex autoimmune disease that can manifest in various ways. There are different types of lupus, each with its own characteristics and symptoms. In this chapter, we will explore the most common types of lupus, including systemic lupus erythematosus, cutaneous lupus, drug-induced lupus, and neonatal lupus.

### ___Systemic Lupus Erythematosus (SLE):___

Systemic lupus erythematosus, often referred to simply as SLE or lupus, is the most common and well-known form of lupus. It is a chronic autoimmune disease that can affect various parts of the body, including the skin, joints, kidneys, heart, lungs, brain, and blood cells. In SLE, the immune system mistakenly attacks healthy tissues and organs, causing inflammation and a wide range of symptoms. Common symptoms include joint pain, skin rashes, fatigue, and fever. The severity of SLE can vary greatly from person to person, and it may flare up intermittently.

### ___Cutaneous Lupus:___

Cutaneous lupus is a subtype of lupus that primarily affects the skin. It may present as various skin problems, such as rashes and lesions, without significant involvement of internal organs. The most common skin manifestations in cutaneous lupus are discoid lupus erythematosus (DLE) and subacute cutaneous lupus erythematosus (SCLE). DLE often results in round, scaly, and raised skin lesions, while SCLE is characterized by reddish, coin-shaped lesions that are often triggered or exacerbated by exposure to sunlight. Cutaneous lupus can occur on its own or coexist with systemic lupus erythematosus.

### ___Drug-Induced Lupus:___

Drug-induced lupus is a form of lupus that is triggered by certain medications. Unlike systemic lupus erythematosus, drug-induced lupus typically resolves when the person stops taking the medication responsible for their symptoms.

Common medications associated with drug-induced lupus include hydralazine, procainamide, and isoniazid. Symptoms of drug-induced lupus are similar to those of SLE and may include joint pain, skin rashes, and fever. This type of lupus is relatively rare compared to SLE.

### *Neonatal Lupus:*

Neonatal lupus is a condition that affects infants born to mothers with certain lupus-specific autoantibodies. These autoantibodies can cross the placenta during pregnancy and affect the baby. The most common manifestation of neonatal lupus is a skin rash that typically appears in the first few weeks of life. Neonatal lupus can also affect the heart, blood, and liver of the baby. Fortunately, most infants with neonatal lupus do not go on to develop SLE, and the condition usually improves within a few months after birth.

It's important to note that these are the main types of lupus, but the disease can affect individuals differently, and there are other less common forms and subsets of lupus as well. Each type of lupus may require different approaches to management and treatment, so it's essential for individuals with lupus to work closely with their healthcare providers to develop a personalized care plan.

***A place to write down your questions, thoughts, and other notes:***

1. +

+

3. +

4. +

5. +

6. +

7. +

"Believe in the power of your dreams, for they are the blueprints of your

reality waiting to be brought to life through your

determination and actions."

- Unknown

***

# CHAPTER 3 PERSONAL NOTES

CHAPTER FOUR

# *Living with Lupus*

- **Coping with the Emotional Impact**

- **Building a Support System**

- **Communicating with Loved Ones**

- **Mental Health and Lupus**

Living with lupus can be challenging, both physically and emotionally. This chapter will address some important aspects of coping with the emotional impact of the disease and how to build a support system to help you navigate this journey. We will also explore the importance of effective communication with loved ones and how mental health plays a significant role in managing lupus.

### *Coping with the Emotional Impact:*

- Understanding Lupus: The first step in coping with the emotional impact of lupus is to educate yourself about the disease. Understanding its symptoms, triggers, and treatment options can help you feel more in control.

- Seeking Emotional Support: Living with a chronic illness like lupus can be emotionally draining. Reach out to support groups, therapists, or counselors who can provide you with the emotional support you need.

- Self-Care: Practice self-care by engaging in activities that relax and rejuvenate you. This might include hobbies, mindfulness exercises, or meditation.

- Acceptance and Grief: It's normal to grieve the life you had before lupus. Allow yourself to process these emotions and work towards accepting your new reality.

- Setting Realistic Goals: Set achievable goals for yourself, both short-term and long-term. This can help you maintain a sense of purpose and control.

### *Building a Support System:*

- Family and Friends: Lean on your close friends and family for support. They can be a crucial part of your support system and offer understanding and empathy.

- Support Groups: Joining a lupus support group can connect you with others who are going through similar challenges. Sharing experiences and advice can be empowering.

- Healthcare Team: Your medical professionals can also be part of your support system. Keep open lines of communication with them, and don't hesitate to ask questions or seek assistance.

- Online Communities: Consider participating in online communities and forums where you can connect with fellow lupus patients. These communities can provide valuable insights and a sense of belonging.

### *Communicating with Loved Ones:*

- Honesty: Be open and honest with your loved ones about your condition. Share your symptoms, needs, and limitations to foster understanding.

- Education: Encourage your family and friends to learn more about lupus. This will help them better grasp what you're going through.

- Setting Boundaries: Establish clear boundaries when necessary. Let your loved ones know when you need rest or help, and don't be afraid to communicate your limitations.

- Expressing Gratitude: Show appreciation for the support you receive. Expressing gratitude can strengthen your relationships and make your support system more willing to help.

### **_Mental Health and Lupus:_**

- Seeking Professional Help: If you're struggling with mental health issues such as depression or anxiety, don't hesitate to seek help from a mental health professional. They can provide therapy or medication if needed.

- Stress Management: Managing stress is crucial for lupus patients. Practice stress-reduction techniques such as yoga, meditation, and deep breathing exercises.

- Medication and Lupus: Some lupus treatments can affect your mental health. Discuss potential side effects with your healthcare team and communicate any concerns.

- Nutrition and Exercise: A balanced diet and regular exercise can have a positive impact on your mental health. Consult your doctor for a suitable exercise plan.

Living with lupus can be challenging, but with the right coping strategies, a strong support system, and attention to your mental health, you can lead a fulfilling life despite the disease. Remember that you are not alone, and there are resources and people available to help you on your journey.

**_A place to write down your questions, thoughts, and other notes:_**

1. +

2. +

3. +

4. +

5. +

6. +

7. +

**"Peace is not merely a distant goal, but a journey of understanding,**

**tolerance, and compassion that begins within each of us."**

**- Linda Fierro**

***

# CHAPTER 4 PERSONAL NOTES

CHAPTER FIVE

---

# *Treatment Options for Lupus*

L upus, a chronic autoimmune disease, can affect various parts of the body, leading to a wide range of symptoms. Treatment for lupus often involves a combination of medications, non-pharmacological treatments, complementary and alternative therapies, and strategies for managing flare-ups.

**Medications for Lupus:**

- **_Nonsteroidal Anti-Inflammatory Drugs (NSAIDs):_** These over-the-counter or prescription drugs can help relieve pain and reduce inflammation associated with mild lupus symptoms, such as joint pain.

-

**_Corticosteroids:_** Prednisone and other corticosteroids can be prescribed to manage more severe symptoms or flare-ups. They work by suppressing the immune system's activity and reducing inflammation.

- **_Antimalarial Drugs:_** Hydroxychloroquine and chloroquine are often used to manage lupus symptoms, particularly skin and joint problems. They can help modulate the immune response.

- **_Immunosuppressants:_** Medications like azathioprine, methotrexate, mycophenolate mofetil, and cyclophosphamide may be prescribed to suppress the immune system's abnormal activity and reduce organ damage.

- **_Biologics:_** Some biologic medications, such as belimumab, specifically target the immune system to manage lupus symptoms.

- **_Monoclonal Antibodies:_** Rituximab is a monoclonal antibody that can target specific immune cells and may be used in certain cases of lupus.

- **_Topical Steroids:_** For skin symptoms, topical steroids in the form of creams or ointments may be used.

**Non-pharmacological Treatments:**

- **_Rest and Exercise:_** Finding the right balance of rest and physical activity is essential for managing lupus.

Regular, gentle exercise can help with joint flexibility and overall well-being.

- **_Diet:_** A healthy, balanced diet can help manage inflammation and maintain overall health. Omega-3 fatty acids, found in fish and flaxseed, may be beneficial. Avoiding excessive salt can help manage fluid retention common in lupus.

- **_Sun Protection:_** Sunlight can trigger lupus flares, so it's essential to use sunscreen, wear protective clothing, and limit sun exposure.

- **_Sleep Management:_** Prioritizing good sleep hygiene can help reduce fatigue, a common symptom of lupus.

**Complementary and Alternative Therapies:**

- **_Acupuncture:_** Some people with lupus find acupuncture to be helpful in managing pain and reducing stress.

- **_Yoga and Tai Chi:_** These gentle, low-impact exercises can improve flexibility and reduce stress, which can benefit individuals with lupus.

- **_Massage Therapy:_** Massage can help relax muscles and reduce pain and stress.

- **_Herbal Supplements:_** Some people turn to supplements like fish oil, turmeric, and probiotics to manage lupus symptoms. Always consult a healthcare professional before trying any alternative therapies.

**Managing Flare-Ups:**

- **_Medication Adjustments:_** During a flare-up, your healthcare provider may adjust your medications to control symptoms more effectively.

- **_Rest:_** It's essential to prioritize rest during a flare-up to allow your body to heal and reduce the risk of exacerbating symptoms.

- **_Stress Management:_** Stress can trigger or worsen lupus symptoms, so stress-reduction techniques like meditation, mindfulness, and relaxation exercises are essential.

- **_Regular Follow-Ups:_** Stay in close contact with your healthcare team for regular check-ups and to monitor your condition.

It's important to work closely with your healthcare team to develop a treatment plan tailored to your specific needs. Lupus management often requires a combination of these treatment options to achieve the best outcomes, and the approach may need to be adjusted over time to address changing symptoms and disease activity.

*A place to write down your questions, thoughts, and other notes:*

1. +

2. +

3. +

4. +

5. +

6. +

7. +

"Strength doesn't come from what you can do; it arises from overcoming

the things you once thought you couldn't."

- Rikki Rogers

***

# CHAPTER 5 PERSONAL NOTES

CHAPTER SIX

# Lifestyle Adjustments

- **Diet and Nutrition**

- **Exercise and Physical Activity**

- **Sleep and Fatigue Management**

- **Coping with Sun Sensitivity**

In this chapter, we will explore various lifestyle adjustments that can help you improve your overall well-being and manage certain health conditions. These adjustments include:

- ***Diet and Nutrition:***

    o

A balanced and healthy diet is essential for maintaining good health. It can help prevent chronic diseases, maintain a healthy weight, and provide the necessary nutrients for your body to function optimally.

- Consider consulting with a registered dietitian or nutritionist to create a personalized meal plan that aligns with your health goals and dietary restrictions.

- Focus on consuming a variety of foods, including fruits, vegetables, whole grains, lean proteins, and healthy fats.

- Limit your intake of processed foods, sugary beverages, and excessive amounts of salt and saturated fats.

- Stay hydrated by drinking plenty of water throughout the day.

- **_Exercise and Physical Activity:_**

  - Regular physical activity is essential for maintaining cardiovascular health, muscle strength, and flexibility.

  - Aim for at least 150 minutes of moderate-intensity aerobic activity or 75 minutes of vigorous-intensity aerobic activity per week.

Incorporate strength training exercises at least two days a week to build and maintain muscle mass.

- Choose activities you enjoy to make exercise a sustainable part of your routine.

- ***Sleep and Fatigue Management:***

  - Quality sleep is crucial for physical and mental health. Aim for 7-9 hours of sleep per night.

  - Create a consistent sleep schedule by going to bed and waking up at the same time each day.

  - Make your sleep environment comfortable, dark, and quiet.

  - Manage stress through relaxation techniques like meditation or deep breathing to improve sleep quality.

  - If you experience chronic fatigue, consult with a healthcare professional to identify and address underlying causes.

- ***Coping with Sun Sensitivity:***

  - Sun sensitivity, or photosensitivity, can be a challenge for individuals with certain medical conditions or skin sensitivities. Protect yourself from excessive sun exposure with the following tips:

o Use a broad-spectrum sunscreen with an SPF of 30 or higher and reapply regularly when exposed to the sun.

o Wear protective clothing, including hats, sunglasses, and long-sleeved clothing.

o Seek shade during peak sunlight hours (usually 10 a.m. to 4 p.m.).

o Stay informed about the UV index and take appropriate precautions.

o Consult with a dermatologist or healthcare provider for guidance on managing your specific sun sensitivity condition.

By making these lifestyle adjustments, you can take proactive steps to enhance your overall well-being and better manage health conditions related to diet, exercise, sleep, and sun sensitivity.

**A place to write down your questions, thoughts, and other notes:**

1. +

+

3. +

4. +

5. +

6. +

7. +

**"Adversity introduces a person to themselves. Embrace the challenge, for**

**within it lies the opportunity to discover your true strength."**

**- Unknown**

***

# CHAPTER 6 PERSONAL NOTES

CHAPTER SEVEN

# Lupus and Relationships

- **Maintaining Healthy Relationships**

- **Explaining Lupus to Others**

- **Balancing Intimacy and Self-Care**

- **Joining Lupus Support Groups**

Living with lupus can have a significant impact on your relationships, both with friends and family, as well as with romantic partners. In this chapter, we'll explore ways to maintain healthy relationships, explain lupus to others, balance intimacy and self-care, and the benefits of joining lupus support groups.

### **Maintaining Healthy Relationships:**

Living with lupus can be challenging, and it's important to maintain healthy relationships to help you through the ups and downs. Here are some tips for doing so:

- *Communication:* Open and honest communication is key. Talk to your loved ones about your condition, your needs, and your limitations. Encourage them to ask questions and share their feelings as well.

- *Set Boundaries:* Understand your physical and emotional limits, and don't be afraid to set boundaries. Let others know when you need rest or when you can engage in activities. Respect your own limitations.

- *Patience and Understanding:* Both you and your loved ones should practice patience and understanding. Lupus symptoms can be unpredictable, so flexibility is important. Your friends and family may need time to adjust to your condition.

- *Support System:* Surround yourself with a supportive network of friends and family who can provide emotional and practical support when needed.

### **Explaining Lupus to Others:**

Explaining lupus to others can be challenging, especially since it's an invisible illness. Here are some tips for effectively communicating about your condition:

- *Educate Yourself:* Before you can explain lupus to others, it's important to educate yourself about the condition. Understand its causes, symptoms, and how it affects your daily life.

- *Keep It Simple:* When explaining lupus, keep it simple and straightforward. You don't need to go into medical details unless someone expresses a genuine interest.

- *Use Analogies:* Comparing lupus to something more familiar can make it easier for others to understand. For example, you could liken it to a faulty immune system that attacks healthy cells.

- *Provide Resources:* Offer informational resources or direct people to credible sources where they can learn more about lupus.

### *Balancing Intimacy and Self-Care:*

Maintaining intimacy in a romantic relationship while managing lupus can be a delicate balance. Here's how to strike that balance:

- *Open Communication:* Discuss your needs and concerns with your partner. Talk about your symptoms and how they affect your daily life and intimacy.

- *Plan Intimate Moments:* Plan intimate activities during times when you typically feel better. This can help ensure you have the energy for them.

- *Self-Care:* Prioritize self-care and listen to your body. If you're not feeling well, it's okay to postpone intimacy. Your partner should understand and support your self-care.

- *Seek Professional Help:* If your relationship is significantly affected by lupus, consider couples counseling to address any challenges that arise.

### **Joining Lupus Support Groups:**

Lupus support groups can be incredibly valuable for both emotional and practical support. Here's why you should consider joining one:

- *Emotional Support:* Connecting with others who understand what you're going through can provide emotional comfort and reduce feelings of isolation.

- *Information Sharing:* Support groups often provide valuable information about managing lupus, treatments, and coping strategies.

- *Empowerment:* Being part of a supportive community can empower you to take control of your health and advocate for yourself.

- *Practical Advice:* Members can share practical tips for living with lupus, such as managing symptoms, dealing with medical appointments, and accessing resources.

In summary, managing relationships when living with lupus requires communication, understanding, and support. Explaining lupus to others in a clear and simple way, balancing intimacy and self-care, and joining lupus support groups can all contribute to your overall well-being and quality of life.

*A place to write down your questions, thoughts, and other notes:*

1. +

2. +

3. +

4. +

5. +

6. +

7. +

**Love: A gentle breeze embracing two souls' dance.**

*"Love is composed of a single soul inhabiting two bodies."*

*- Aristotle*

***

# CHAPTER 7 PERSONAL NOTES

## CHAPTER EIGHT

---

# Managing Work and Lupus

- **Navigating Workplace Challenges**

- **Requesting Accommodations**

- **Career Planning and Long-Term Goals**

- **Financial Management**

Living with lupus can present unique challenges when it comes to managing work and pursuing a career. In this chapter, we will discuss various aspects of managing work and lupus, including how to navigate workplace challenges, requesting accommodations, career planning and setting long-term goals, and managing your finances while living with this autoimmune disease.

### *Navigating Workplace Challenges:*

Living with lupus may mean dealing with symptoms like fatigue, joint pain, and flares. These challenges can affect your ability to work effectively. Here are some strategies to help you navigate workplace challenges:

- *Open Communication:* Communicate with your supervisor or HR department about your lupus diagnosis. This can help them better understand your needs and make accommodations if necessary.

- *Flexible Work Arrangements:* Consider flexible work hours or telecommuting options to help manage your symptoms and work more comfortably.

- *Balancing Rest and Work:* It's important to find the right balance between work and rest. Listen to your body and take breaks when needed.

- *Self-Advocacy:* Advocate for yourself and your health. Be open about your limitations and educate colleagues about lupus to reduce stigma.

### *Requesting Accommodations:*

The Americans with Disabilities Act (ADA) provides legal protection for individuals with disabilities, including lupus. You may request reasonable accommodations to help you perform your job more effectively. Common accommodations for lupus may include:

- *Flexible hours:* Adjust your work schedule to accommodate times when you feel your best.

- *Ergonomic workspace:* Modify your workspace to reduce physical strain and discomfort.

- *Reduced workload:* Adjust your workload during flares or when symptoms are particularly severe.

- *Assistive technology:* Use technology that helps with tasks that may be difficult due to lupus-related challenges.

### **Career Planning and Long-Term Goals:**

Despite lupus, you can still plan for a successful career. Here are some tips:

- *Set Realistic Goals:* Consider your limitations and set achievable career goals.

- *Continued Education:* Explore opportunities for skill development and education to enhance your qualifications.

*Networking:* Build a professional network to access support and opportunities.

- *Financial Planning:* Consider long-term financial goals and how your career choices can help you achieve them.

## *Financial Management:*

Managing your finances while living with lupus is essential to maintain stability and meet your healthcare needs. Here are some financial management tips:

- *Budgeting:* Create a budget that considers medical expenses, insurance, and day-to-day living costs.

- *Health Insurance:* Ensure you have adequate health insurance to cover lupus-related expenses.

- *Emergency Fund:* Build an emergency fund to cover unexpected medical bills or work disruptions.

- *Disability Benefits:* Investigate if you are eligible for disability benefits or other financial assistance.

- *Legal Support:* Consider seeking legal advice regarding financial matters if necessary.

Managing work and lupus can be challenging, but with proper strategies and support, you can navigate these challenges successfully. Open communication, self-advocacy, and a realistic approach to career planning can help you achieve your long-term goals while managing your health and financial needs.

***A place to write down your questions, thoughts, and other notes:***

1. +

2. +

3. +

4. +

5. +

6. +

7. +

**Hope: Radiant dawn after the darkest night's embrace.**

*"Hope is being able to see that there is light despite all of the darkness."*

*- Desmond Tutu*

***

***

# CHAPTER 8 PERSONAL NOTES

CHAPTER NINE

---

# *Pregnancy and Lupus*

- **Fertility and Lupus**

- **Preconception Planning**

- **Pregnancy and Lupus Flares**

- **Postpartum Care**

**<u>*Fertility and Lupus:*</u>**

- *Fertility Concerns:* Women with lupus may have concerns about their fertility. While lupus itself doesn't necessarily impact fertility, certain medications used to manage lupus, like cyclophosphamide, may affect fertility. It's essential to discuss fertility preservation options with your healthcare provider if you plan to have children.

### *Preconception Planning:*

- *Consultation with a Rheumatologist:* Women with lupus should consult with a rheumatologist before planning a pregnancy. This helps in assessing the readiness of the individual's lupus for pregnancy and ensuring that the condition is stable.

- *Medication Review:* Review and adjust lupus medications to minimize potential risks during pregnancy. Some medications may need to be adjusted or discontinued to reduce potential harm to the fetus.

- *Overall Health Optimization:* Focus on overall health, including controlling disease activity, maintaining a healthy diet, exercising, and managing stress.

- *Vaccinations:* Ensure that vaccinations are up-to-date as some vaccines may not be safe during pregnancy.

- *Supplement Consideration:* Folic acid supplements may be recommended to prevent birth defects.

### *Pregnancy and Lupus Flares:*

- *Disease Flare Risk:* Pregnancy can affect lupus in various ways. Some women may experience a lupus flare during pregnancy, especially during the first trimester and shortly after childbirth.

- *Monitoring:* Close monitoring by healthcare providers is crucial to detect and manage any flare-ups promptly.

- *Medication Management:* Medication regimens may need to be adjusted during pregnancy to balance disease control and safety for the baby.

- *High-Risk Pregnancy:* Women with lupus may be considered high-risk pregnancies, and they may need more frequent prenatal check-ups and specialized care.

### *Postpartum Care:*

- *Continued Monitoring:* After giving birth, monitoring and care for both the mother and the baby should continue. Lupus flares can occur in the postpartum period.

- *Breastfeeding Consideration:* Some lupus medications may not be safe during breastfeeding. Consult with your healthcare provider to determine the best approach for you.

- *Family Planning:* Discuss future family planning, including birth control options, with your healthcare provider.

This information is a general overview, and specific recommendations will vary depending on the individual's unique circumstances and the severity of their lupus.

**A place to write down your questions, thoughts, and other notes:**

1. +

2. +

3. +

4. +

5. +

6. +

7. +

**Dreams: Ambitions soaring beyond the horizon's grasp.**

*"The future belongs to those who believe in the beauty of their dreams."*

*- Eleanor Roosevelt*

***

# CHAPTER 9 PERSONAL NOTES

CHAPTER TEN

# Research and Emerging Treatments

- **Advances in Lupus Research**

- **Clinical Trials and Participation**

- **Potential Future Therapies**

- **Advocacy and Awareness**

In recent years, there have been significant advancements in lupus research, offering hope for improved treatments and, ultimately, a cure for this autoimmune disease. This chapter will delve into the latest developments in lupus research, the importance of clinical trials and patient participation, potential future therapies on the horizon, and the role of advocacy and awareness in the fight against lupus.

### *Advances in Lupus Research:*

- *Understanding the Immune System:* Researchers have made substantial progress in comprehending the complex immune system dysregulation in lupus. They have identified specific immune cells and molecules that play key roles in the disease, such as B cells and interferons.

- *Genetics:* Genetic research has revealed a strong genetic component in lupus, and specific risk genes have been identified. Understanding the genetic basis of lupus can lead to targeted therapies and personalized medicine approaches.

- *Environmental Triggers:* Researchers are investigating environmental factors that can trigger lupus in genetically predisposed individuals, such as infections, UV radiation, and hormonal changes.

- *Biomarkers:* The search for reliable lupus biomarkers has intensified. Biomarkers can aid in diagnosis, disease monitoring, and the development of targeted therapies.

### *Clinical Trials and Participation:*

- *Importance of Clinical Trials:* Clinical trials are essential for evaluating the safety and efficacy of potential lupus treatments. They provide an opportunity for patients to access cutting-edge therapies and contribute to advancing medical science.

- *Phases of Clinical Trials:* Clinical trials typically progress through four phases, from safety testing to large-scale effectiveness studies. Each phase provides critical information about a treatment's benefits and risks.

- *Patient Participation:* Patient involvement in clinical trials is crucial. Patients can join clinical trials through their healthcare providers and advocacy organizations. Participation helps researchers collect data and refine treatments.

## *Potential Future Therapies:*

- *Biologics:* Biologic drugs that target specific molecules involved in the immune response show promise in treating lupus. Monoclonal antibodies, for example, can block harmful immune signals.

- *Small Molecule Inhibitors:* These drugs can block or modulate certain cellular pathways involved in lupus, potentially reducing disease activity and flares.

- *Stem Cell Therapy:* Stem cell transplantation is a potential option for severe lupus cases. It involves resetting the immune system to reduce autoimmune activity.

*Precision Medicine:* The future of lupus treatment may involve personalized approaches based on genetic and biomarker information. This could lead to more effective and tailored therapies.

### ***Advocacy and Awareness:***

- *Patient Advocacy Groups:* Various lupus advocacy organizations work to raise awareness, provide support, and advocate for research funding. These groups empower patients to engage in their healthcare and contribute to lupus research.

- *Education and Awareness Campaigns:* Public awareness about lupus is crucial to reduce stigmatization and promote understanding. Education campaigns can help people recognize symptoms, seek timely diagnosis, and support those living with lupus.

- *Legislation and Policy:* Advocacy efforts aim to influence healthcare policy, increase research funding, and improve access to care for people with lupus.

In conclusion, ongoing research is shedding light on the underlying mechanisms of lupus, leading to potential breakthroughs in treatment. Clinical trials, patient participation, and advocacy are pivotal in this journey. Raising awareness and supporting research can improve the quality of life for those affected by lupus and may eventually lead to a cure.

**A place to write down your questions, thoughts, and other notes:**

1. +

2. +

3. +

4. +

5. +

6. +

7. +

**Courage: The fearless heart in the face of adversity's roar.**

*"Courage is not the absence of fear,*

*but the triumph over it."*

*- Nelson Mandela*

***

# CHAPTER 10 PERSONAL NOTES

CHAPTER ELEVEN

---

# Thriving with Lupus

- **Setting Goals and Expectations**

- **Monitoring Your Health**

- **Embracing a Positive Mindset**

- **Inspiring Lupus Success Stories**

Living with lupus can be challenging, but it's possible to thrive and lead a fulfilling life. In this chapter, we'll explore some key strategies for thriving with lupus, including setting goals and expectations, monitoring your health, embracing a positive mindset, and finding inspiration in lupus success stories.

***Setting Goals and Expectations:***

Living with lupus requires careful planning and goal-setting. It's essential to set realistic and achievable goals that take your health and limitations into account. Consider both short-term and long-term goals, and be flexible in adapting them as your health fluctuates. Some goals to consider might include:

- *Health and Symptom Management:* Set goals for managing your lupus symptoms, such as reducing pain, fatigue, and inflammation through medication, lifestyle changes, and holistic approaches like diet and exercise.

- *Daily Living:* Establish goals for maintaining daily routines and activities, such as work, household chores, and social interactions, while considering your energy levels and limitations.

- *Emotional Well-being:* Focus on goals related to emotional well-being, such as stress management, anxiety reduction, and building a support network of friends and family.

### **Monitoring Your Health:**

Regularly monitoring your health is crucial for managing lupus effectively. This includes working closely with your healthcare team to track your symptoms, medications, and overall well-being. Consider these practices:

- *Keep a Symptom Journal:* Maintain a journal to record your symptoms, their severity, and any triggers or patterns you notice. This information can be invaluable during medical appointments.

- *Medication Management:* Ensure you take your prescribed medications as directed and keep track of any side effects or changes in your condition. Communicate openly with your healthcare provider about any concerns.

- *Regular Check-Ups:* Schedule regular check-ups with your rheumatologist or specialist to monitor your disease activity and discuss treatment adjustments as needed.

### Embracing a Positive Mindset:

Maintaining a positive mindset is essential when dealing with a chronic illness like lupus. Consider these strategies:

- *Self-Care:* Prioritize self-care, including adequate rest, a balanced diet, regular exercise (as approved by your healthcare provider), and stress management techniques.

- *Mindfulness and Meditation:* Practicing mindfulness and meditation can help reduce stress and improve your mental outlook. These techniques can also assist in managing pain and fatigue.

- *Support Networks:* Build a support network of friends, family, and support groups. Sharing your experiences and challenges with others who understand can be a source of encouragement and inspiration.

### ***Inspiring Lupus Success Stories:***

Reading or listening to success stories of people who have thrived with lupus can be highly motivating. These stories often highlight the importance of resilience, adaptability, and determination in the face of adversity. You can find inspiration from various sources, including books, blogs, podcasts, and support groups where individuals share their journeys.

Remember that thriving with lupus is a personal journey, and it may involve trial and error as you discover what works best for you. Be patient with yourself, adapt to changes in your health, and stay committed to your goals and well-being. By setting realistic expectations, monitoring your health, maintaining a positive mindset, and drawing inspiration from others, you can lead a fulfilling life despite lupus.

***A place to write down your questions, thoughts, and other notes:***

1. +

2. +

3. +

4. +

5. +

6. +

7. +

**Faith: Unseen wings lifting souls to limitless heights.**

*"Faith is taking the first step even when you don't see the whole staircase."*

*- Martin Luther King Jr.*

***

# CHAPTER 11 PERSONAL NOTES

***

You are welcome to check out my new website @ https://My-Lupus-Journey.com

I always enjoy your thoughts, so please comment on my website, or you can

email me @ MyLupusJourney777@gmail.com

Stay Positive and know that each moment is a true Blessing for all of us.

***